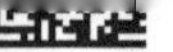

Copyright 2023

Table of Contents

PREVIEW 4

MACROBIOTIC DIET RECIPES 6

BREAKFAST 6

1. Vegan Panini with Marinated Tofu and Avocado 6

2. Crock Pot Baked Apples 8

3. Lemon Blueberry Baked Oatmeal 9

4. Vegan Chocolate Chip Zucchini Muffins 11

5. Chocolate Oatmeal 13

6. Healthy Carrot Cake Oatmeal 15

7. Homemade Refried Beans 16

8. Healthy Strawberry Crumble 18

9.Avocado Mango Salad Bowl 20

10. Grilled Vegan Caesar Salad with Crispy Tofu Croutons 22

LUNCH 25

11. Chickpea Quinoa Salad With Marinated Tomatoes 25

12. Tahini Pasta 27

13. Savory Oatmeal With Pan-Seared Tofu 29

14. Vegan Gnocchi Tomato Soup 32

15. Peanut Miso Chickpea Salad Stack 34

16. Roasted Sweet Potato Quinoa Salad With Sesame Miso
Sauce 36

17. Lemon Garlic Marinated Chickpea Wraps 39

18.15 Minute Garlic Sesame Noodles 41

19. Zesty Lime Marinated Black Bean Bowl 43

20. Vegan Pesto Sandwich with Crispy Herb Tofu 45

DINNER 47

21. Citrus Infused Couscous Chickpea Salad 47

22. Buffalo Tofu Wraps 49

23. Dominican Spiced Mashed Chickpea Salad.............................. 51

24. Chickpea Quinoa Salad with Marinated Tomatoes 53

25. Cucumber Boats with Crispy Chickpeas................................ 55

26. Greek-Inspired Chickpea Tofu Wraps.................................. 57

27. Garlic Chili Tofu with Peanut Sauce 59

28. Mustard Chili Chickpeas 61

29. Tofu and Lentil Curry 63

30. Mango Coconut Chickpea Curry 65

PREVIEW

Macrobiotic diets combine the concepts of Buddhist spirituality and certain dietary principles with the goal of balancing spiritual and physical wellness. Macrobiotic diets aim to avoid the "toxins" that come from eating dairy products, meats, and oily foods. A macrobiotic diet consists largely of whole grains, cereals, and cooked vegetables.

The macrobiotic diet is low in meat and low in other foods that are high in zinc. Milk products are a good source of zinc for those who consume them. Zinc absorption from plant foods is poor when the foods contain phytate and oxalate inhibitors. Macrobiotic diets are high in foods high in the zinc inhibitor phytic acid (e.g., soy products, beans, lentils, peas, nuts, and whole grains). Good plant sources of zinc are zinc-fortified cereals, and yeast-fermented foods that reduce the phytic acid content of whole-grain breads, rather than refined white bread. Zinc supplements are also good sources of zinc that may be acceptable to some macrobiotics. Fermented soyfoods, like tempeh and miso, and sprouted legumes may have more bioavailable zinc than unfermented foods like tofu and soymilk.

The main advantage of the Macrobiotic diet is the cleansing that happens to the body of all stored up toxins, excess fat and even stored up dark/sad emotions. It is a very sattvic diet that helps you keep a calm mind and soul. It heals illnesses without medicines or needing very little medication. Macrobiotic diet is very popular with cancer patients as they are usually recommended high fiber and low fat foods.

Vegetables, beans and whole grains in the macrobiotic diet guarantee high fiber and low fat content, thus avoiding high fat and saturated fat. There is also the presence of phytoestrogens in this diet with soyfood and this is known to mitigate the menstrual problems that bother women most often.

Many nutritionists believe the macrobiotic diet—especially the one propagated by George Ohsawa is a very restrictive diet. The diet is stepped up in different stages and at once stage the practitioner is allowed only brown rice and water. Avoidance of dairy food in the diet leads to a severe calcium deficiency that is compensated through nuts and green leafy vegetables, only to a certain extent.

MACROBIOTIC DIET RECIPES

BREAKFAST

1. Vegan Panini with Marinated Tofu and Avocado
Prep Time: 10 Minutes

Cook Time: 20 Minutes

Servings: 3

Ingredients

- 1 block (450g) extra firm tofu, pressed and drained
- 1/4 cup soy sauce
- 1 tbsp apple cider vinegar
- 1 tbspdijon mustard
- 2 tbsp maple syrup
- 1 tsp Italian seasoning
- 1 tsp garlic powder
- 1 tsp oregano
- 1 tsp cornstarch or nutritional yeast

Sandwich Assembly

- 1 cup mushrooms, sliced
- 1 small onion, cut into slices
- 1 medium avocado, mashed, or sub vegan cheese
- 6–8 slices of Sprouted Soft Wheat Bread
- 2 handfuls of baby spinach, optional
- 2 tbsp vegan butter
- 1 tsp miso paste

Instructions

1. Marinade the tofu. Cut your tofu into thin slabs. In a large airtight container, mix together all the remaining marinade ingredients. Place tofu in the marinade, seal the container and give a gentle shake to make sure the tofu is coated. Allow to sit for a few minutes while you heat your panini grill and prepare your other ingredients. Place the tofu onto the heated gridle and cook the tofu for 2-3 minutes then flip to cook on the other side.
2. Prepare the vegetables. Add your mushrooms and onions to a heated non-stick skillet to cook down with a pinch of salt and pepper until most of the moisture from the mushrooms has cooked off and the onions have softened.
3. Prepare the sandwich. To a slice of bread, mash on a thin layer of avocado along with a pinch of salt and pepper. Top the avocado with the spinach, then the tofu slices, followed by the mushrooms and onions. Mix together some vegan butter and miso to spread on the other piece of toast.
4. Cook the sandwich. Place the toast with the butter mixture facing the outside of the sandwich, then place the sandwich butter side down on the griddle. Spread some of the butter mixture on the top slice of the bread facing you and then close the griddle down between your sandwich. Gently press down to help seal the sandwich and allow to cook for about 2 minutes or until you get some nice grill marks. Then, serve your sandwich immediately.

2. Crock Pot Baked Apples
Prep Time: 15 Minutes

Cook Time: 2hrs 2 Minutes

Servings: 6

Ingredients

- 3 pounds Fuji Apples, peeled and sliced thin or cubed based on preferences
- Juice of one lemon, about 2 tbsp
- 1 tbsp organic brown sugar
- 1 tbsp cornstarch
- 1 tsp cinnamon
- 1/4 tsp cardamom
- 1/4 tsp Chinese 5 spice or a pinch of freshly grated nutmeg

Instructions

1. Place all your apples in the slow cooker and toss with the remaining ingredients to coat.
2. Cover your slow cooker with a lid and set to high and cook for 1 ½ hours to 2 hours, stirring occasionally as the apples cook down to your liking (stirring 1-2 times is plenty).
3. Serve on top of your oats as a quick way to jazz up your oats in the morning or on top of toast with peanut butter.

3. Lemon Blueberry Baked Oatmeal

Prep Time: 10 Minutes

Cook Time: 40 Minutes

Servings: 4

Ingredients

- 2 tbsp ground flax seeds
- 4 tbsp water
- 1 cup gluten-free rolled oats
- 1/2 cup gluten-free quick oats
- 2 tsp baking powder
- 1/2 tsp salt

Juice and zest of one lemon

- 1/3 cup almond or cashew butter
- 1/3 cup maple syrup
- 1 tsp vanilla extract
- 1/2 tsp almond extract or 1 extra tsp of vanilla extract
- 1 1/4 cups almond milk

Blueberry Jam

- 1 cup frozen blueberries
- 1 tbsp maple syrup, optional
- 1/2 tsp cornstarch

Lemon Yogurt Drizzle

- 1/4 cup vegan unsweetened yogurt
- Extra lemon zest and 1/2 tbsp lemon juice
- 1 tbsp maple syrup or more to sweeten to preference

Instructions

1. Heat up a small sauce pan and add in your frozen blueberries and maple syrup. Stir until the blueberries have released their juices and thawed. Stir in your cornstarch and continue to stir for an additional 2 minutes to help them thicken, then remove from heat. They will continue to thicken as they cool.
2. Set oven to 350F. In a small bowl combine your flax seed and water and allow to gel for 5 minutes as you prepare the remaining ingredients.
3. To a medium sized bowl, add in your rolled oats, quick oats, baking powder, salt and lemon zest. Give everything a good mix to combine.
4. To the dry ingredients, add in the nut butter, maple syrup, lemon juice, extracts, flax egg and almond milk. Give everything another mix until everything is well combined.
5. Pour the batter into a lightly greased 9-in x 9-in baking dish. Drop dollops of blueberry jam over the surface of the batter and gently swirl overtop (do not overmix).
6. Place the baking dish in the oven for 40 minutes. The oats should be golden and the center of the oatmeal should appear set and firm. If jiggly, bake for an additional 5 minutes.
7. As the oats cool out of the oven, prepare the yogurt drizzle by combining all the ingredients in a small bowl until smooth. When serving, pour your lemon yogurt overtop your oatmeal slice and enjoy.

4. Vegan Chocolate Chip Zucchini Muffins
Prep Time: 20 Minutes

Cook Time: 23 Minutes

Servings: 12

Ingredients

- 1 cup One Degree Organics Sprouted Gluten-Free Rolled Oats
- 1 cup unsweetened plant-based milk of choice
- 1 1/2 cups whole wheat pastry flour, white wheat flour or all-purpose flour
- 1/2 cup coconut sugar or organic light brown sugar
- 2 tsp baking powder
- 1 tsp baking soda
- 1/2 tsp salt
- 2 tsp ground cinnamon
- 1/4 tsp nutmeg
- 1/4 cup unsweetened apple sauce
- 1 tbsp apple cider vinegar
- 1 cup zucchini, grated
- 1 tsp vanilla extract
- 1/2 cup or more dairy-free chocolate chips

Instructions

1. Set the oven to 425F and prepare your muffin pan by either spraying with non-stick spray or lining with muffin liners and set aside.

2. Add your oats and milk to a bowl and allow to soak for 20 minutes. Measure and prep your remaining ingredients as you wait.
3. To a separate bowl, add in your flour, sugar, baking soda, baking powder, cinnamon, nutmeg and salt and give a good mix to combine.
4. In the same bowl, add in your apple sauce, apple cider vinegar, vanilla extract, zucchini and your soaked oats.
5. Mix your ingredients together to form a thick batter, then fold in your chocolate chips.
6. With a cookie scoop or spoon, divide your batter evenly into your muffin tin. Then place your muffins into the oven.
7. Bake your muffins at 425F for 5 minutes and while keeping the muffins in the oven, reduce the heat to 350F and continue baking for an additional 18 minutes or until a toothpick pierces the center and comes out clean. Allow to fully cool then enjoy.

5. Chocolate Oatmeal
Prep Time: 5 Minutes

Cook Time: 15 Minutes

Servings: 2

Ingredients

- 1/2 cup raw hazelnuts (optional)
- 1/2 cup gluten-free rolled oats
- 1/2 cup gluten-free quick oats
- 1/4 cup Dutch-processed cocoa powder
- 1 tbsp ground flaxseed
- 1/4–1/2 tsp salt, based on preference
- 2 tbsp nut or seed butter (I used peanut butter)
- 2–3 tbsp maple syrup or organic brown sugar or coconut sugar (use what you like to sweeten)
- 2 cups unsweetened almond milk
- Serve With
- Dairy-Free Dark Chocolate Chips
- Fruit like banana or raspberries

Instructions

1. Set oven to 350F. To a lined baking sheet add the hazelnuts and place in the oven to roast for 10-12 minutes. Remove from the oven and allow to cool as you prep your oats.
2. To a saucepan add your remaining oatmeal ingredients and bring to a low simmer, stirring regularly until the oats thicken to your liking, about 3-5 minutes.

3. Remove the cooked oats from heat. Now, rub the hazelnuts between your palms to remove any excess skins that flake off. Portion your oats and top with chocolate chips, hazelnut and fruit for the ultimate experience.

6. Healthy Carrot Cake Oatmeal

Prep Time: 5 Minutes

Cook Time: 10 Minutes

Servings: 3

Ingredients

- 1 cup grated carrot, about 2 medium carrots
- 1 cup gluten-free rolled oats
- 1/2 tsp ground ginger
- 1 1/2 tsp cinnamon
- 1/2 tsp allspice
- 1/2 cup unsweetened apple sauce
- 2 cups unsweetened almond milk
- 2 tbsp maple syrup or brown sugar, optional or to taste
- 1 tsp vanilla extract
- 1/4 cup raisins
- 1/4 cup walnuts, chopped
- 1/4 tsp salt or more to taste

Instructions

1. Add all the ingredients to a sauce pan and stir to combine.
2. Bring the oats to a simmer while stirring frequently to help the oatmeal thicken. Cook for about 5-8 minutes or until the oatmeal is slightly underdone to your thickness preference.
3. Remove from heat and let it sit then top with extra toppings as desired and serve.

7. Homemade Refried Beans

Prep Time: 5 Minutes

Cook Time: 1hr 15 Minutes

Servings: 6

Ingredients

- 1 cup dry black beans
- 1 small white or yellow onion, cut in half and save 1/2 for the boiled beans and dice up the other half for the refried beans
- 7 cloves of garlic, crush 1 clove for the refried beans
- 1 bay leaf
- 2 tbsp olive oil
- 1 jalapeño or serrano pepper, seeds removed if desired
- 1/2 vegetable bouillon cube or 1/2 tsp Vegetable or Vegan Chicken Better than Bouillon
- Salt to taste

Instructions

If Cooking Beans From Scratch

1. Measure your beans then spread out on a sheet pan and sort, removing any extra debris, rocks or shriveled or broken pieces. Rinse the beans well and place the beans in a large pot with enough water to reach 3 inches above the beans.
2. Add in 1/2 your onion, 6 cloves of garlic and your bay leaf. Bring the pot to a boil over medium-high heat, then simmer the beans and loosely cover the pot with a lid. Cook the beans for 2-3 hours or until the beans

are tender. As the beans cook, stir occasionally and add additional hot water as needed, I often will add about 2 cups of extra hot water to the pot after an hour and a half. After cooking, add salt to taste.
3. Refried Beans
4. Heat up a large skillet on the stove top, add your oil and when hot add in the onion with a pinch of salt and cook down until softened. Then, if using jalapeño, add to the pan and sauté until the jalapeno starts to sear, about 2-3 minutes.
5. Add 3 cups of cooked beans with bean liquid OR 2, 15 oz cans of black beans with their liquid to the pan and mix in with the onion mixture. As the beans simmer, add in the bouillon base and use a potato masher to mash up the beans.
6. Continue to cook the beans until a nice puree forms. You can leave it as chunky as you like.

8. Healthy Strawberry Crumble
Prep Time: 15 Minutes

Cook Time: 40 Minutes

Servings: 6

Ingredients

Strawberry Filling

- 2 lbs fresh strawberries, quartered (about 5 cups)
- 2 tbsp maple syrup or agave
- Juice of half a lemon
- 1 tbsp cornstarch
- Oat Crumble
- 1 cup One Degree Organics Sprouted Rolled Oats
- 5 tbsp almond flour, oat flour or all-purpose flour
- 1/2 cup walnuts, chopped
- 1/2 tsp cinnamon
- 1/3 cup maple syrup
- 1/3 cup almond butter or peanut butter
- 1/2 tsp almond extract or 1 tsp vanilla extract
- Pinch of salt

Instructions

1. Preheat your oven to 350F. Add your chopped strawberries to fill the entire bottom of an 8-in x 8-in ceramic baking pan.
2. Top the strawberries with cornstarch, maple and lemon juice and then toss together to combine making

sure the cornstarch is mostly dissolved by the juiciness of the strawberries.

3. In a separate bowl, add your remaining dry ingredients and mix together with a fork. Pour in the almond butter and maple syrup and mix making sure your dry and liquid ingredients are fully combined.
4. Top your strawberries with the crumble and bake in the oven for 40 minutes.
5. After cooking, remove the baking dish from the oven and allow to set for about 15-20 minutes before serving.

9.Avocado Mango Salad Bowl
Prep Time: 10 Minutes

Cook Time: 10 Minutes

Servings: 4

Ingredients

- 2 cups frozen edamame, thawed
- 2 ataulfo mangos, pitted and cubed
- 2 avocados, pitted and cubed
- 1/2 a small red onion, about 1/4 cup diced
- 1/3 cup cilantro, minced
- 1–2 limes
- 1 tbsp soy sauce
- 2 tsp maple syrup or agave
- 1/2 tbsp or more of chili crisp oil or 1/2 tbsp toasted sesame oil
- 2 cloves garlic, minced
- 2 cups shishito peppers or bell peppers of your choice, stems removed and roughly chopped
- Oil for sauteing
- Salt and pepper to taste

Instructions

1. To a mixing bowl add in your edamame, mango, avocado, red onion, cilantro, and the zest of 1 lime.
2. Add a small sprinkle of salt and the juice of 2 limes over top along with your soy sauce, sweetener, and chili oil. Give the salad a good mix and let it sit and marinade as you prepare the shishito peppers.

3. To a skillet over medium-low heat, add a splash of oil. Once warmed through, add in your garlic and sauté until fragrant. Add the peppers and continue to sauté until the peppers start to brown, about 3 minutes.
4. Add a small sprinkle of salt and then add the peppers and garlic to avocado mango mix and stir to combine. Serve as a nutritious power bowl with some cooked rice, extra greens and more toppings like chili oil as desired.

10. Grilled Vegan Caesar Salad with Crispy Tofu Croutons

Prep Time: 15 Minutes

Cook Time: 19 Minutes

Servings: 4

Ingredients

Tofu Croutons

- 1 (454g) package of Nasoya Super Firm Tofu, cut into cubes
- 1 tbsp cornstarch
- 1 tbsp nutritional yeast
- 1 tbsp gluten-free soy sauce or coconut aminos
- 1 tbsp olive oil
- 1 tsp garlic powder
- 1 tsp onion powder
- 1 tsp Italian seasoning

Creamy Tahini Caesar Dressing

- 1/3 cup good quality tahini
- 2 garlic cloves, crushed
- Juice and zest of 1/2 a large lemon
- 2 tsp capers + 2 tbsp of juice from the caper jar
- 1 tsp Dijon mustard
- 1 tsp vegan Worcestershire sauce, optional
- 3 tbsp nutritional yeast
- 1/4 cup cold water

Grilled Romaine Lettuce

- 3 heads Romaine lettuce heads, cut in half lengthwise

- 2 tbsp olive oil

Juice and zest of half a large lemon

- 1 clove garlic, crushed
- Salt and pepper to taste

Instructions

1. For the tofu: Place your cubed tofu in a medium sized mixing bowl. Top the tofu with the cornstarch, nutritional yeast, soy sauce, oil, garlic powder, onion powder and Italian seasoning. Give the tofu a toss to coat and place in your air fryer to bake at 390F for 17 minutes until browned and crispy.
2. Prepare the Caesar dressing: To a bowl or large measuring cup add in the tahini, garlic, lemon juice and zest, capers and caper juice, mustard, Worcestershire sauce, and nutritional yeast and whisk together to combine. When the dressing starts to thicken, slowly whisk in the water until the dressing is your desired consistency.
3. Grill the Romaine Lettuce: To a small bowl combine the olive oil, zest, juice, garlic and a few cracks of salt and pepper and mix well. Brush this oil mixture overtop the cut side of the Romaine head and bring to a preheated grill. Place the Romaine cut side down on the grill and allow to cook for 1-2 minutes or until the bottoms are browned or appear to develop grill marks. Remove the lettuce and set aside on a platter to assemble your salad.
4. Assemble: Use 1/2 a head of lettuce per serving and plate it with a generous serving of the dressing and

top with the tofu croutons. Adjust and add more salt
and pepper to taste and serve.

LUNCH

11. Chickpea Quinoa Salad with Marinated Tomatoes
Prep Time: 10 Minutes

Cook Time: 20 Minutes

Servings: 3

Ingredients

- 1 cup dry quinoa, rinsed
- 2 cups vegetable broth (or 2 cups water with a vegetable bouillon cube)
- 1 cup cherry tomatoes, halved
- 2 cloves garlic, crushed and divided
- 1 shallot, minced
- 3 tbsp fresh parsley, minced
- 3 tablespoons extra virgin olive oil
- 1 1/2 tbsp balsamic vinegar
- 1/4 tsp red pepper flakes, optional
- 1 tsp sugar or maple syrup, optional
- 1, 15 oz can chickpeas, rinsed and drained

Zest and juice of one small lemon

- 1 tsp dry oregano
- 2–3 Persian cucumbers or 1/2 an English cucumber, chopped
- 1/4 cup marinated artichoke hearts, chopped
- 1 cup frozen corn, thawed
- 1/4 cup fresh basil leaves
- Salt & pepper

Instructions

1. To cook the quinoa, add it to a large sauce pan along with 2 cups of vegetable broth. Bring the quinoa to a boil and then immediately reduce the heat to the lowest setting then cover. Cook the quinoa covered for 15 minutes and remove from heat and allow to stand for 5-10 minutes with the lid on. Remove the cover, fluff and stir then allow the quinoa to sit for an extra 5-10 minutes uncovered.
2. In a small bowl add in the halved tomatoes and sprinkle with a pinch of salt and pepper. Add one garlic clove that's been crushed, shallot, parsley, 2 tablespoons extra virgin olive oil, balsamic vinegar, and pepper flakes. Give everything a good mix, taste and if the vinegar is strong add the sugar and mix again then set aside.
3. Add your drained chickpeas to a bowl and add the remaining garlic, zest, lemon juice, oregano and a good pinch of salt and pepper. Mix again and set aside with the tomatoes for 15 minutes.
4. To a large mixing bowl add in your quinoa, cucumbers, artichoke hearts, corn, and basil leaves. Top with the marinated chickpeas and tomatoes making sure to drizzle on top any of the remaining dressing from the tomatoes. Toss together and serve.

12. Tahini Pasta
Prep Time: 10 Minutes

Cook Time: 20 Minutes

Servings: 6

Ingredients

Tahini Pasta Sauce

- 1/3 cup good quality tahini
- 2 tbsp nutritional yeast, optional
- 2 tbsp extra virgin olive oil, divided
- 1 tsp Italian seasoning
- 1 tsp yellow or white miso paste, optional

Juice and zest of one medium lemon

- 1 tsp maple syrup
- Salt and Pepper
- 1/4 cup ice water to thin

Assemble

- 1 lb pasta, I used rigatoni
- 1 shallot, sliced
- 4 cloves garlic, minced
- 1 bunch of kale, stems removed
- 1 cup reserved pasta water
- 1/4 cup parsley, minced
- 1/4 cup Basil leaves, sliced

Instructions

1. Tahini Sauce: Mix the tahini, 1 tablespoon of olive oil, nutritional yeast, Italian seasoning, miso paste, lemon, maple syrup, and a good pinch of salt and pepper together until it starts to thicken. Slowly pour in the the iced cold water and whisk until no lumps remain in the sauce.
2. Pasta: Bring a pot of water to a boil and generously salt it. Once boiling add the pasta and cook according to package. Reserve some pasta water, then drain the pasta.
3. Assemble: To a large skillet heat the remaining olive oil then sauté your shallots until softened. Stir in the garlic and continue sauteing until fragrant. Add the kale and sauté until it has wilted. To the pan, add in the warm pasta, the tahini sauce and the reserved pasta water. Give the pasta a good mix to coat. Top with some minced parsley, fresh basil leaves, fresh cracked black pepper and salt and extra lemon zest before serving.

13. Savory Oatmeal with Pan-Seared Tofu

Prep Time: 15 Minutes

Cook Time: 25 Minutes

Servings: 3

Ingredients

Pan Seared Tofu

- 1, 450g block extra firm tofu, drained and pressed for 15 minutes
- 1 tbsp gluten-free soy sauce or tamari
- 1 tbsp nutritional yeast
- 1 tbsp cornstarch
- 1 tbsp avocado oil

Oatmeal

- 1 tsp avocado oil
- 1 scallion, thinly sliced
- 1 1/2 cups water
- 1 cup unsweetened soy milk
- 4 shiitake mushrooms
- 1 tbsp soy sauce
- 1 cup One Degree Organics Gluten-Free Sprouted Rolled Oats
- 1 tsp chili garlic sauce
- 1 tbsp yellow miso paste
- 2 cups curly kale, roughly chopped and stems removed
- Serving
- Avocado Slices
- Chili Oil

- Sesame Seeds

Instructions

1. Cut your tofu into cubes or triangles. Add the tofu to an airtight container along with cornstarch, nutritional yeast, salt and pepper. Seal the container and give a few gentle shakes to evenly coat the tofu.
2. Heat up a large skillet over medium heat and then add your oil to warm through. Once the oil is hot, add in your tofu making sure to spread them out into a single layer in the pan to cook. Allow the tofu to cook undisturbed for about 4 minutes. Flip and cook on the opposite side for an additional 3-4 minutes or until the tofu has become golden. Remove the tofu and place on a plate with a clean paper towel and set aside.
3. To prepare the oatmeal, heat a saucepan over medium-low heat and add a drizzle of oil. When the oil is hot, add the white portion of the sliced scallion with a pinch of salt and sauté for 2 minutes until softened.
4. Add in the milk, water, soy sauce and the dry shiitake mushrooms. Stir the mixture well and bring to a simmer.
5. Remove and reserve the mushrooms from the broth. Add your miso paste to a small bowl and pour over about 3 tablespoons of the warm milk mixture over the miso then mix to break up any clumps. Pour this mixture back into the saucepan along with the oats and chili garlic sauce.
6. Stir the mixture frequently as it comes back to a simmer and allow to cook for 3-5 minutes or until the

oats start to thicken. Add the kale and allow it to cook down and wilt into the oats. Continue to cook until the oats have thickened to your liking then serve. If desired, slice the rehydrated mushrooms to use on top of the oats along with a few pieces of tofu, sliced avocado, scallions, chili oil and sesame seeds.

14. Vegan Gnocchi Tomato Soup
Prep Time: 10 Minutes

Cook Time: 30 Minutes

Servings: 6

Ingredients

- 1–2 tsp avocado oil
- 1 medium yellow onion, diced
- 1 red bell pepper, diced
- 1/4 cup sun-dried tomatoes, diced
- 6 garlic cloves, crushed
- 1 tbsp tomato paste
- 2 tsp smoked paprika
- 1/2 tsp fennel seeds
- 1/4–1/2 tsp red pepper flakes, optional
- 1, 15 oz can of chickpeas, rinsed and drained
- 1, 15 oz can crushed tomatoes
- 5 cups of vegetable broth
- 1/4 cup nutritional yeast
- 6 sprigs of fresh thyme, stems removed
- 1 cup vegan cashew cream or canned coconut milk (for cashew cream soak 3/4 cup raw cashew in hot water for 30 minutes, discard liquid and blend cashews with 1/4 cup water with a pinch of salt until smooth)
- 1 package (~500g) of shelf stable gnocchi
- 2 cups kale, roughly chopped
- 3 tbsp fresh parsley, roughly chopped
- Salt and pepper to taste

Instructions

1. Heat a large pot over medium heat, then add oil to warm through. Add in the onions along with a pinch of salt and sauté until the onions has softened and become translucent.
2. Add in the bell pepper and sun-dried tomatoes and continue to sauté for 2 minutes to help the bell pepper soften.
3. Stir in the garlic, cooking until it becomes fragrant, then add in the tomato paste. Cook the paste for 2-3 minutes before adding in the smoked paprika, fennel, and red pepper flakes and continue to stir and sauté for an extra minute to combine.
4. Add in the chickpeas and stir to coat. Pour in the crushed tomatoes, vegetable broth, nutritional yeast and thyme. Stir well to combine, bring to a simmer and then cover and cook for 15 minutes.
5. Pour in the vegan cream, gnocchi, kale and parsley then stir well and allow to to cook according to the recommended cooking time for the gnocchi. Once cooked, taste and adjust with salt and pepper to taste before serving topped with more fresh herbs as desired.

15. Peanut Miso Chickpea Salad Stack
Prep Time: 20 Minutes

Cook Time: 00 Minutes

Servings: 4

Ingredients

Peanut Miso Chickpea Salad

- 1, 15 oz can of chickpeas, rinsed and drained
- 2 tbsp peanut butter
- 2 tsp yellow miso paste
- 1 tbspsriracha
- 2 tsp maple Syrup
- 1 tbsp rice wine vinegar

To Assemble Bowl or Stack

- 2 cups cooked Brown Rice
- 1 avocado, mashed
- 1 cucumber, thinly sliced
- 1/2 cup shredded carrots

Sesame Seeds

- Soy Sauce or Coconut Aminos
- Sesame oil or spray oil

Instructions

1. To prepare the chickpeas, place in a medium sized mixing bowl and mash to your desired consistency with a fork.

2. Add in your peanut butter, sriracha, miso paste, maple syrup, and vinegar and continue to mix well to combine making sure to mash the miso well so no large clumps remain.

3. If you wish to season your rice, combine 2 cups cooked brown rice with 2 tbsp rice wine vinegar, 1 tsp of cane sugar and 1 tbsp of sesame seeds in a bowl. Mix well then set aside.

4. To assemble your stack, start by spraying or rubbing the inside of a large measuring cup or flat bottom cup with sesame oil. Now layer the cucumber slices so that they cover the bottom of your cup. Add 2 tbsp or more of mashed avocado and spread it evenly to coat the layer of cucumber. Add 1/4 cup of your mashed chickpea mixture, then fill the remainder of the cup with rice making sure it is pressed and smoothed evenly into the cup.

5. Run a thin knife along the edges of the cup to help make releasing the stack easier. Place a flat bottom plate on top of the stack and then carefully flip. You may need to carefully tap the top of the cup to release the contents. Lift the cup away and you should be left with a stack. If any of the cucumber pieces get stuck to the cup, just carefully remove them and place on top of your stack.

6. To serve, drizzle with a little soy sauce or sesame oil then top with some sesame seeds and scallions if desired.

16. Roasted Sweet Potato Quinoa Salad with Sesame Miso Sauce

Prep Time: 15 Minutes

Cook Time: 35 Minutes

Servings: 4

Ingredients

- 1 cup dry quinoa, rinsed and drained
- 2 cups vegetable broth
- 1 large sweet potato, cut into 3/4 inch pieces
- 1 1/2 cups broccoli florets, about 1 medium head
- 1, 15 oz can of chickpeas, rinsed, drained and pat dry with a clean towel
- 1 tbsp avocado oil
- 2 tsp chili garlic sauce
- 2 tsp maple syrup
- 1/2 tsp ground ginger
- 1 tsp garlic powder
- Salt

Sesame Miso Sauce

- 4 tbsp tahini
- 1 tbsp yellow or white miso paste
- 1 tbsp gluten-free soy sauce
- 2 tbsp rice vinegar
- 1/2 tsp ground ginger
- 1 tsp garlic powder
- 2 tsp maple syrup
- 2 tsp sesame oil
- 2–3 tbsp water

Assembly

- 2 scallions, finely sliced
- 1/4 cup cilantro, finely diced
- 2 tsp gluten-free soy sauce
- 2 tsp sesame oil
- Sesame seeds

Instructions

1. Add the quinoa to a large sauce pan with vegetable broth and a pinch of salt. Bring the quinoa to a boil, reduce the heat to a simmer and cover with a lid. Let it cook for 15 minutes, remove from heat and sit for 5 minutes then fluff with a fork. Once cooked set aside.
2. Preheat oven to 375F. To a large sheet pan add the sweet potatoes and chickpeas. To another sheet pan add the broccoli.
3. Whisk together the oil, chili sauce, maple syrup, ginger and garlic in a bowl then drizzle it over the potatoes, chickpeas and broccoli. Toss everything to coat and spread everything out on a single layer to roast evenly on their respective sheet pans.
4. Sprinkle the trays with a pinch of salt and place the potatoes and chickpeas in the oven to bake for 20 minutes. Give the potatoes a flip and toss the chickpeas and return back to the oven along with the tray of broccoli and roast for 10-15 minutes or until the potatoes are fork tender.

5. Make the sesame tahini sauce by whisking all the listed sauce ingredients together until smooth. If too thick, thin out with 1-2 extra tbsp of water.
6. To a large mixing bowl add the quinoa, potato, chickpeas, broccoli, cilantro, scallions, soy sauce, sesame oil and a pinch of salt. Toss to coat. Plate and serve with dressing and sesame seeds.

17. Lemon Garlic Marinated Chickpea Wraps
Prep Time: 15 Minutes

Cook Time: 00 Minutes

Servings: 8

Ingredients

- 2, 15 oz cans of chickpeas, rinsed and drained
- 1 cup cucumber, diced
- 1 cup cherry tomatoes, quartered
- 1/4 cup red onion, finely diced
- 1/4 cup fresh parsley, finely chopped
- 2 tbsp fresh mint or basil, finely chopped
- 2 tbsp extra virgin olive oil
- 1 tsp Dijon mustard

Juice and zest of 1 medium lemon

- 1 tbsp apple cider vinegar
- 2 cloves garlic, crushed
- 1/2 tsp dry oregano
- 1/2 tsp dry thyme
- 1/2 tsp dry basil
- 2 tsp maple syrup or agave
- Salt
- Serve With
- Whole Grain Pitas or Wraps
- Hummus or Lemon Garlic White Bean Spread

Instructions

1. To a large mixing bowl add in the chickpeas, cucumbers, tomatoes, red onion, parsley and mint then sprinkle with a pinch of salt.
2. In a separate jar add in the oil, mustard, apple cider vinegar, garlic, oregano, thyme, basil, maple syrup and a pinch of salt. Give the dressing a really good mix to combine then pour it over the chickpea mixture.
3. Toss the chickpea salad together, making sure it has been coated with the dressing then cover the bowl and place in the fridge for up to one hour, stirring occasionally to redistribute the dressing.
4. When ready to serve, place a wrap or pita on a flat plate and spread with your favorite spread then top with the chickpea salad and serve.

18.15 Minute Garlic Sesame Noodles
Prep Time: 15 Minutes

Cook Time: 00 Minutes

Servings: 3

Ingredients

Noodle Bowl

- 4 oz of brown rice vermicelli noodles
- 1 1/2 cups frozen edamame, thawed
- 1/2 cup or more shredded carrot
- 1/2 cup or more shredded cabbage
- 1/2 cup or more julienned or shredded Persian cucumber
- 1 tbsp toasted sesame seeds (serve as is or grind in a mortar and pestle)
- Sauce
- 2 tbsp tahini or sesame paste
- 2 tbsp natural peanut butter, with salt
- 2 tbsp gluten-free soy sauce or coconut aminos
- 1 tbsp rice wine vinegar
- 1 tbsp maple syrup or 2 tsp sugar
- 1 tbsp vegan mayo (optional)
- 1/2 tbsp sesame oil
- 1/2 tbsp or more chili oil (for less spicy replace with more sesame oil)
- 1–2 cloves garlic, finely grated
- 1/2 inch fresh ginger, finely grated
- 2 to 4 tbsp of water

For Serving, Optional

- Fresh minced cilantro and/or mint
- Sliced scallions
- Lime wedges
- Baked Tofu or store bought pre-cooked tofu

Instructions

1. Bring a tea kettle with water to a boil. Place the noodles in a medium mixing bowl and pour over the noodles and cover to allow them to soak and rehydrate. When rehydrated according to package, drain off the excess water and set aside.
2. Prepare the sauce by combining the tahini, peanut butter, soy sauce, vinegar, syrup, sesame oil, chili oil, garlic and ginger in a small bowl and give a good mix until it starts to clump. Slowly pour in 2 tablespoons of water then mix together. Add additional water 1 tablespoon at a time until desired creamy consistency is achieved. Make sure to taste the sauce and adjust the amount of garlic, soy sauce, chili oil, etc. to your liking.
3. Assemble to serve by adding a serving of the noodles to a plate topped with the shredded vegetables and thawed edamame. Then pour over with the sesame sauce and garnish with fresh herbs, scallions and the toasted sesame seeds.

19. Zesty Lime Marinated Black Bean Bowl
Prep Time: 15 Minutes

Cook Time: 00 Minutes

Servings: 6

Ingredients

Bean Bowl Base

- 2, 15 oz cans of black beans, rinsed and drained
- 1 1/2 cups frozen fire roasted corn, thawed
- 1 red bell pepper, diced
- 1/4 cup diced red onion, about half a small onion
- 1 cup cherry tomatoes, halved
- 1/4 cup fresh cilantro, minced
- Tortillas or Tortilla chips for serving
- Lime Dressing
- Juice and zest of 2 limes
- 2 tbsp extra virgin olive oil
- 2 tbsp apple cider vinegar or white wine vinegar
- 1 tbsp maple syrup or agave, adjust amount based on preference
- 2 cloves garlic, crushed
- 1/2 tsp ground cumin
- 1–2 tsp smoked paprika, chipotle powder or chili powder
- 1/4 tsp salt or more to taste
- Optional Topping Ideas
- Pickled Jalapenos
- Pickled Onions
- Vegan Sour Cream

- Salsa Verde
- Shredded Cabbage

Instructions

1. To a large mixing bowl add in the black beans, cherry tomatoes, red onion, bell pepper, and cilantro then sprinkle with a pinch of salt.
2. In a separate jar or to the same bowl add in the lime zest and juice, oil, apple cider vinegar, maple syrup, garlic, cumin, smoked paprika, and a pinch of salt. If combining separately, give the dressing a really good mix then pour it over the black bean mixture.
3. Toss the black beans and dressing together, making sure it has been coated with the dressing then cover the bowl and place in the fridge for up to one hour, stirring occasionally to redistribute the dressing.
4. When ready to serve, place a wrap or pita on a flat plate and spread with your favorite spread then top with the chickpea salad and serve.

20. Vegan Pesto Sandwich with Crispy Herb Tofu
Prep Time: 5 Minutes

Cook Time: 25 Minutes

Servings: 4

Ingredients

Crispy Tofu

- 1 tbsp nutritional yeast
- 1 tbsp cornstarch
- 1/2 tsp garlic powder
- 1/2 tsp thyme
- 1 tbsp soy sauce
- 1 tbsp avocado oil
- 1 block (450g) extra firm tofu, drained and pat dry with a kitchen towel then cut into 4 length sized slabs

To Assemble Sandwich

- 1 large ripe tomato, I used an heirloom and cut into slices
- 1–2 cups baby spinach
- 2 slices of hearty whole grain bread per sandwich (can make up to 4 sandwiches)
- 1–2 tbsp of dairy-free red pesto or store bought pesto per sandwich
- Salt

Instructions

1. To a shallow dish add your nutritional yeast,
   cornstarch, garlic, thyme and give a good mix to
   combine. Pour in the oil and soy sauce and mix again
   into a wet batter.
2. Pat your tofu dry with a clean kitchen towel and cut
   the block into 4 slabs lengthwise. Take each tofu slab
   and coat evenly in the batter. Place the tofu in an air
   fryer basket and then cook at 400F for 15 minutes.
3. Spread pesto on both slices of bread and then layer
   one slice with the spinach, the crispy tofu, and a slice
   or two of tomatoes. Sprinkle the tomatoes with a
   pinch of salt and then close the sandwich with the
   other slice of bread spread with pesto.
4. If toasting your sandwich, place the sandwich in a
   panini press to warm through on both sides. Cook
   until golden on both sides, about 5-6 minutes (See
   notes for cooking without a panini press).

DINNER

21. Citrus Infused Couscous Chickpea Salad
Prep Time: 15 Minutes

Cook Time: 00 Minutes

Servings: 4

Ingredients

Citrus Infused Couscous Chickpea Salad

- 1 cup dry couscous
- 1 cup hot water
- 2 Persian cucumbers, sliced or diced
- 1 bell pepper, diced
- 1/3 cup fresh parsley, minced
- 2 tbsp fresh mint, minced
- 1/4 cup canned mandarin oranges, packed in juice
- 1/4 cup sliced almonds
- 1/4 cup chopped dates, raisins, or craisins
- 1, 15 oz can chickpeas, rinsed and drained

Dressing

- 2 shallots, thinly sliced
- 3 cloves garlic, crushed
- Zest and juice of 1 lemon
- Zest and juice of 1 lime
- Juice of 1 small orange
- 1 tbsp white wine vinegar
- 1 tbsp maple syrup, optional
- 1/2 tsp Chinese 5 Spice
- Pinch of salt

Instructions

1. Add the couscous and hot water to a bowl. Mix and then cover with a lid and let stand for10 minutes until all the water is absorbed.
2. Combine all the dressing ingredients in a large mug or jar and give it a good mix to combine.
3. Fluff the couscous with a fork then top with the chopped vegetables, canned and dried fruit, chickpeas, herbs, almonds and a generous pinch of salt.
4. Pour over the dressing. Mix everything together and add more salt and pepper if needed then serve.

22. Buffalo Tofu Wraps

Prep Time: 10 Minutes

Cook Time: 25 Minutes

Servings: 3

Ingredients

Buffalo Tofu

- 1, 450g block extra firm tofu, pressed and drained
- 2 tbsp soy sauce or coconut aminos
- 1 tbsp avocado oil
- 2 tbsp cornstarch
- 1 tsp thyme
- 1/4 tsp black pepper
- 1/4 cup vegan buffalo sauce

To Assemble

- Vegan Ranch
- Shredded Lettuce
- Flatbread, Pita or Gluten-Free Wraps
- Sliced Scallions
- Parsley
- Buffalo Tahini Sauce
- 2 tbsp tahini
- 5–6 tbsp of hot sauce
- 1 tbsp maple syrup
- 1 tbsp apple cider vinegar
- 1/2 tbsp soy sauce
- Juice of half a small lemon
- Tahini Ranch Sauce

- 2 tbsp tahini
- 1 tbsp vegan plain unsweetened yogurt
- 1/2 tbsp apple cider vinegar
- Juice of half a lemon
- 1/2 tsp garlic powder
- 1 tsp dry dill
- Pinch of salt
- 1–2 tbsp water to thin to your liking

Instructions

1. Preheat your oven to 425F. In a bowl, break up your tofu into 1 inch chunks and coat with the soy sauce, oil, cornstarch, thyme and pepper and toss to coat.
2. Place the tofu on a lined baking sheet and bake in the oven for 25 minutes making sure to flip halfway through.
3. If making the recommended homemade sauces, do so while the tofu is baking. Prep your buffalo tahini sauce and tahini ranch sauce separately in different jars. Mix both until completely smooth.
4. Once the tofu is baked and crispy, add your baked tofu to a bowl and toss with the Buffalo sauce to coat.
5. To assemble your pita, spread your vegan ranch overtop, add on the shredded lettuce, a few spoons of the buffalo tofu and any extra sauce you like. Sprinkle with herbs and scallions and enjoy.

23. Dominican Spiced Mashed Chickpea Salad
Prep Time: 15 Minutes

Cook Time: 00 Minutes

Servings: 3

Ingredients

Mashed Chickpea Salad

- 1, 15 oz can chickpeas, rinsed and drained
- 2 cloves garlic
- 3 tbsp good quality tahini
- 1/2 tsp adobo seasoning
- 1/2 tspsazon or 1 tsp smoked paprika
- 1/2 tsp oregano
- 1/4 tsp dry thyme
- 1/2 tsp better than bouillon vegetable base or 1/2 veggie bouillon cube
- 1/2 small red onion, finely diced
- 1 bell pepper, finely diced
- 3 tbsp Spanish Olives, minced
- 1/4 cup cilantro, minced
- 1/4 cup parsley, minced
- Juice of 1 lime
- 1 tbsp apple cider vinegar
- 1 tbsp water
- For Sandwich
- 6 slices of whole grain bread
- Mashed avocado
- Tomato slices
- Plantain Chips

- Vegan Ketchup Mayo
- Salt and pepper to taste

Instructions

1. In a bowl add in your chickpeas and mash them to your liking. Add in the garlic, tahini, spices and bouillon then mix together until fully combined.
2. Stir in the diced onion, bell pepper, herbs, lime juice, apple cider vinegar, and water. Mix well until the mixture starts to clump together. Taste and adjust seasonings based on preference.
3. To assemble the sandwich, mash avocado on to one slice of bread then top with the mashed chickpea salad mixture, fresh tomato slices, and plantain chips. Spread some vegan ketchup mayo on the other piece of bread and use it to top the sandwich before enjoying.

24. Chickpea Quinoa Salad with Marinated Tomatoes

Prep Time: 10 Minutes

Cook Time: 20 Minutes

Servings: 3

Ingredients

- 1 cup dry quinoa, rinsed
- 2 cups vegetable broth (or 2 cups water with a vegetable bouillon cube)
- 1 cup cherry tomatoes, halved
- 2 cloves garlic, crushed and divided
- 1 shallot, minced
- 3 tbsp fresh parsley, minced
- 3 tablespoons extra virgin olive oil
- 1 1/2 tbsp balsamic vinegar
- 1/4 tsp red pepper flakes, optional
- 1 tsp sugar or maple syrup, optional
- 1, 15 oz can chickpeas, rinsed and drained
- Zest and juice of one small lemon
- 1 tsp dry oregano
- 2–3 Persian cucumbers or 1/2 an English cucumber, chopped
- 1/4 cup marinated artichoke hearts, chopped
- 1 cup frozen corn, thawed
- 1/4 cup fresh basil leaves
- Salt & pepper

Instructions

1. To cook the quinoa, add it to a large sauce pan along with 2 cups of vegetable broth. Bring the quinoa to a boil and then immediately reduce the heat to the lowest setting then cover. Cook the quinoa covered for 15 minutes and remove from heat and allow to stand for 5-10 minutes with the lid on. Remove the cover, fluff and stir then allow the quinoa to sit for an extra 5-10 minutes uncovered.
2. In a small bowl add in the halved tomatoes and sprinkle with a pinch of salt and pepper. Add one garlic clove that's been crushed, shallot, parsley, 2 tablespoons extra virgin olive oil, balsamic vinegar, and pepper flakes. Give everything a good mix, taste and if the vinegar is strong add the sugar and mix again then set aside.
3. Add your drained chickpeas to a bowl and add the remaining garlic, zest, lemon juice, oregano and a good pinch of salt and pepper. Mix again and set aside with the tomatoes for 15 minutes.
4. To a large mixing bowl add in your quinoa, cucumbers, artichoke hearts, corn, and basil leaves. Top with the marinated chickpeas and tomatoes making sure to drizzle on top any of the remaining dressing from the tomatoes. Toss together and serve.

25. Cucumber Boats with Crispy Chickpeas
Prep Time: 10 Minutes

Cook Time: 30 Minutes

Servings: 4

Ingredients

- 1, 15 oz can chickpeas, rinsed and drained (you can also use cooked lentils or edamame)
- 1 tbsp avocado oil
- 1/2 tsp each onion powder
- 1/2 tsp garlic powder
- 1/2 tsp smoked paprika
- 1/4 tsp Old Bay Seasoning
- Salt & Pepper
- 1 English cucumber
- 1 cup cooked rice of choice (I used both white rice and black rice)
- Garnish: sliced scallions and cilantro
- Spicy Garlic Tahini Sauce
- 3 tbsp good quality tahini
- 1 tbsp reduced sodium soy sauce or coconut aminos
- 1 tbsp rice wine vinegar
- 2 tsp maple syrup (adjust to taste)
- 2 tsp chili garlic sauce or sriracha
- 3 tbsp cold water

Instructions

1. Preheat your oven to 375F. Place your chickpeas in a clean kitchen towel and pat them dry. Transfer the

chickpeas to a parchment lined baking sheet and drizzle with the oil, onion powder, garlic powder, paprika, Old Bay Seasoning and a pinch of salt and pepper. Toss the chickpeas to evenly coat and then spread them out in a single layer on the tray. Place in the oven to bake for 30 minutes.

2. Prepare the sauce by combining the tahini, soy sauce, vinegar, maple syrup, and chili garlic sauce in a small bowl. Whisk together until the sauce starts to thicken significantly, then slowly pour your water in while whisking. Add additional water 1 tablespoon at a time as needed until the sauce is to your desired pouring consistency.

3. To assemble, cut your cucumber lengthwise and then cut in half again at the width to get 4 equal boat shaped pieces. To help the cucumber lay flat, shave or peel a portion of the bottom of the cucumber so it can lay flat. Deseed the cucumber with a spoon and then stuff each boat with 2-3 spoons of rice. Wet your hands and press the rice into the cucumber so it lays flat. Press the roasted chickpeas into the rice and then drizzle on the tahini sauce. Garnish with minced cilantro and scallions and enjoy.

26. Greek-Inspired Chickpea Tofu Wraps

Prep Time: 20 Minutes

Cook Time: 00 Minutes

Servings: 3

Ingredients

Marinated Chickpea Salad

- 1, 15 oz can chickpeas, rinsed and drained
- 1 bell pepper, diced
- 1/4 medium red onion, finely diced
- 1/2 cup cherry tomatoes, halved
- 3 tbsp kalamata olives, whole or halved
- 1 Persian cucumber, roughly chopped
- Zest and juice of half a lemon
- 2 tsp dry oregano
- 1/2 tsp red pepper flakes, optional
- 2 tsp red wine vinegar
- 2 tsp maple syrup, optional
- Salt & Pepper
- 1 clove garlic, crushed
- 3/4 cup Marinated Tofu or 1/3 cup Vegan Feta
- To Assemble
- 3 wraps of choice
- 1 cup salad greens
- 6 tbsp Vegan Tzatziki, hummus or avocado
- Vegan Tzatziki, optional
- 1 Persian cucumber, about 1/4 cup grated
- 1/2 cup plain unsweetened plant-based yogurt
- 1/2 tbsp or more lemon juice

- 1 clove garlic, crushed
- 2 tbsp dill, minced
- 1/2 tbsp extra virgin olive oil
- Salt

Instructions

1. To a bowl combine all of the chickpea salad ingredients along with a nice pinch of salt and pepper to a large mixing bowl and give a good mix to combine. Allow the chickpeas to marinate for at least an hour before using. **To save time chopping, use a food chopper.
2. If making Tzatziki, grate your other cucumber and then scoop up the shredded cucumber in your hand and gently squeeze the excess liquid out. Place the grated cucumber in a separate bowl along with the remaining tzatziki ingredients. Whisk to combine and adjust salt to taste.
3. Assemble wrap. Smear your wrap with 2 tablespoons of your desired spread (tzatziki, hummus or avocado), add your greens, top with the chickpea salad and marinated tofu or feta. Roll it up and enjoy.

27. Garlic Chili Tofu with Peanut Sauce
Prep Time: 20 Minutes

Cook Time: 60 Minutes

Servings: 3

Ingredients

- Baked Garlic Chili Tofu
- 1 block extra firm tofu, drained and pressed for at least an hour
- 2 tbsp tamari
- 1 tbsp nutritional yeast
- 2 tsp chili garlic sauce
- Peanut Sauce
- 3 tbsp natural peanut butter
- 2 tbsp tamari
- 1 tbsp maple syrup
- 1 tspsriracha
- 1 tsp mustard
- 1/4 tsp garlic powder
- 1/4 tsp ginger powder
- Juice of half a lime
- 2–3 tbsp water

Instructions

For Baking Garlic Chili Tofu

1. Set oven to 400F. After pressing tofu, cut tofu into even cubes and place in a bowl or Tupperware container.

2. Add in remaining ingredients. If using a bowl, lightly toss all ingredients together with a spatula. If using a Tupperware container or zip lock freezer bag, seal container and gently shake contents to evenly coat tofu.
3. Remove tofu and place on a lined baking sheet making sure tofu cubes are not touching.
4. Place in oven for at least 25 minutes or until edges have browned. Remove from oven and set aside.

For Peanut Sauce

1. Add all ingredients to a bowl and whisk together until smooth.

2. Adjust consistency of sauce to your liking by adding additional water in small amounts to achieve desired consistency.

Assemble Bowl

1. Divide tofu and prepared sides between 3 serving bowls or containers.
2. Add tofu along with sides to a bowl and pour about 2 tbsp worth of peanut sauce over top each bowl and toss together. Add more peanut sauce if desired.

28. Mustard Chili Chickpeas
Prep Time: 5 Minutes

Cook Time: 15 Minutes

Servings: 4

Ingredients

- 1 small onion (diced)
- 1 green bell pepper (diced)
- 1 stalk celery (diced)
- 4 cloves garlic (minced)
- 2 tbsp soy sauce
- 1/2 tsp adobo seasoning
- 1 tspsazón (or an extra tsp of chili powder)
- 2 tsp chili powder
- 1/2 tsp smoked paprika
- 2 cans chickpeas (rinsed and drained)
- 2 tsp brown mustard
- 1/4 cup vegetable broth or water
- 2 tsp sugar or maple syrup
- Salt and pepper to taste

Instructions

1. Heat a medium sized pan over medium heat, add diced onion, bell pepper and celery.
2. Sauté to vegetables, allowing onion to become translucent, about 2-3 minutes.
3. Add in garlic and sauté for 1 minute until fragrant.
4. Sprinkle in seasonings and sauté for 1 minute then stir in soy sauce.

5. Then, add chickpeas and mustard and sauté to coat.
6. Finally, add sugar and broth and stir to combine.
7. Bring mixture to a simmer for about 8-10 minutes or until chickpeas are coated in a glossy finish. Taste and then decide if you wish to adjust salt and pepper as desired.

29. Tofu and Lentil Curry
Prep Time: 15 Minutes

Cook Time: 30 Minutes

Servings: 6

Ingredients

- 1/2 medium red onion, diced
- 1/2 green bell pepper, diced
- 1 small sweet potato, cubed
- 3 cloves garlic, minced
- 1 inch ginger, minced
- 1 tbsp tomato paste
- 1 tbsp curry powder
- 1 tsp cumin
- 2 tsp smoked paprika
- 1 15 oz can diced fire roasted tomatoes
- 1 cup green lentils
- 1 cup light or full fat coconut milk
- 1 block super firm tofu, cubed
- 1 1/2 cups vegetable broth

Instructions

Stove Top Instructions

1. Heat up your pan to medium heat and saute onion and green peppers until onion is translucent.
2. Add in sweet potato, ginger and garlic and make sure to continue moving them around the pan to prevent them from burning.

3. Add tomato paste along with spices and saute until fragrant, about 1-2 minutes.
4. Stir in lentils, diced tomatoes, coconut milk, give a good stir to fully combine.
5. Gently fold in tofu along with vegetable broth. Bring mixture to a boil and then immediately reduce to a low simmer and allow to cook for 25-30 minutes or until lentils are tender.

Instant Pot Instructions

1. Set Instant Pot to saute. Follow all instructions as you would if cooking on stove top.
2. Once you've added the vegetable broth, switch Instant Pot to manual high pressure. Set timer to 13 minutes and make sure lid is set to seal.
3. Allow pressure to release naturally. Remove lid and serve curry as desired.

30. Mango Coconut Chickpea Curry
Prep Time: 15 Minutes

Cook Time: 20 Minutes

Servings: 6

Ingredients

- 1 small onion, diced
- 5–6 cloves garlic, minced
- 2 inch piece of fresh ginger, minced
- 1 tbsp tomato paste
- 1 tbsp curry powder
- 1 tsp garam masala
- 2 cans chickpeas, rinsed and drained
- 2 cups chopped cauliflower florets
- 2 cans lite coconut milk
- Juice and zest of 1 lime
- 1 cup mango, diced
- 1 tbsp maple syrup (optional)
- Salt to taste

Instructions

1. In a large non-stick sauce pan or pot, add onion and sauté until softened. If you use oil, add a small amount to prevent sticking.
2. Add in ginger, garlic, tomato paste, curry powder and Garam masala. Stir and sauté for a minute or until fragrant.

3. Add in cauliflower and a splash of coconut milk and sauté an extra minute then add in chickpeas and remainder of coconut milk.
4. Stir together and bring to a simmer. Simmer on low heat for 10 minutes.
5. Add in mango, stir and cook for another 3-5 minutes or until curry has thickened.
6. Remove from heat and add the lime juice and zest.
7. Stir, add salt to taste and/or sweetener as desired and serve.